An Essential

Guide to Renal Diet

A Pragmatic Approach to Keep your Weight and Kidney Function in Check with Quick & Easy Recipes for Newly Diagnosed

Hayden Johnson

TABLE OF CONTENTS

INTRODUCTION 6

BREAKFAST 9

1. Apple Sauce Cream Toast 9
2. Waffles 11
3. Egg Whites and Veggie Bake 13
4. Peach Berry Parfait 15
5. Open-Faced Bagel Breakfast Sandwich 16
6. Bulgur Bowl with Strawberries and Walnuts 17
7. Overnight oats three ways 19

LUNCH 21

8. Chicken with Quinoa and Wild Rice 21
9. Pineapple and Mint Lamb Chops 23
10. Maple-Brined Pork Loin 24

DINNER 26

11. Falafel 26
12. Israeli Pasta Salad 28
13. Artichoke Matzo Mina 30
14. Sautéed Chickpea and Lentil Mix 32

MAIN DISHES 34

15. Quinoa & Veggie Croquettes 34

16. Salmon Burgers 36

SNACKS 37

17. Parmesan quinoa with peas 37

18. Mushroom orzo 39

19. Carrot and pineapple slaw 41

20. Sesame cucumber salad 42

SOUP AND STEW 44

21. Stuffed bell pepper soup 44

22. Italian chicken stew 46

23. Turkey pasta stew 48

24. One-pot chicken pie stew 50

25. Spring Veggie Soup 52

VEGETABLE 55

26. Crack Slaw 55

27. Vegan Chili 57

28. Chow Mein 59

29. Mushroom Tacos 61

SIDE DISHES 62

30. Chicken and Mandarin Salad 62

SALAD 63

31. Italian Cucumber Salad 63

32. Grapes Jicama Salad 64

FISH & SEAFOOD 65

33. Spanish Tuna 65

34. Fish with Vegetables 67

35. Creamy Crab over Salmon 69

36. Curried fish cakes 71

37. Baked sole with caramelized onion 73

POULTRY RECIPES 75

38. Grilled Chicken with Pineapple & Veggies 75

39. Ground Turkey with Veggies 77

40. Ground Turkey with Asparagus 78

41. Ground Turkey with Peas & Potato 80

MEAT RECIPES 82

42. Beef Brochettes 82

43. Country Fried Steak 84

BROTHS, CONDIMENT AND SEASONING 86

44. Salsa Verde 86

45. Grape Salsa 88

46. Apple and Brown Sugar Chutney 89

DRINKS AND SMOOTHIES 90

47. Honey Cinnamon Latte 90

48. Cinnamon Smoothie 92

DESSERT 93

49. Smooth Coffee Mousse 93

50. Almond Bites 95

51. Bacon Bell Peppers 96

52. Corn & Carrot Fritters 97

53. Butter Baked Nuts 99

54. Eggs Spinach Side 101

55. Squash and Cumin Chili 103

56. Fried Up Avocados 105

57. Hearty Green Beans 106

58. Parmesan Cabbage Wedges 107

59. Extreme Zucchini Fries 108

60. Easy Fried Tomatoes 110

INTRODUCTION

You can build your own meals by being imaginative with leftover food to make perfect fast lunches with oil. Nothing beats vegetarian food for keeping the kidneys safe, but this low-salt kidney-friendly recipe, which has been approved by a kidney dietitian for diets with chronic kidney disease, is a good place to start. Kidney nutrition of vegetables: A vegetarian diet is the only way to keep your kidneys safe. The kidneys need as much protein as possible in their normal diet, and they are made up of all essential amino acids.

Patients with kidney disease can follow the kidney dietary recommendations to the letter, but following a kidney disease diet to the letter can be difficult. This list of kidney diets and meals will make your life and that of your family much simpler. It can be difficult to keep track of a kidney disorder. Strictly - A kidney disease diet can be difficult to follow, which is why we've put together this list of kidney nutrition and kidney disease foods. This kidney nutrition and menu lists would make it easy for you and your family.

It can be tough to stick to a kidney disease diet. A kidney disease diet can be difficult to follow, but this rundown of kidney nutrition and meals can make it simpler for you and your family.

Here's a list of tasty dinners and recipes with a kidney failure diet, as well as a diet to endorse a kidney-friendly dialysis diet. For your family and friends, you'll find recipes for tasty meals, nutritious snacks, and kidney-friendly diets here. You'll find nutritious snacks and menus for you and your friends and family here, as well as a healthy kidney diet schedule. Balanced meals and nutritional foods for the kidney will also be available, as well as healthy foods and nutrition for kidney disease.

Here's an example of a week's worth of meal planning to help you better consider what you should and should eat. This is a compilation of tasty kidney-friendly dialysis menus, as well as nutritious snacks and diets for kidney failure patients.

The following kidney nutrition recipes are ideal for people with kidney disease because they contain few foods that encourage inflammation and other problems, such as sugar and processed carbs, which promote inflammation and other problems. They're also good for people who don't have kidney failure because they don't contain a lot of food that causes inflammation or other issues. Here's a rundown of the kidney dietary recommendations, as well as a look at the sugar consumption for diabetes. The following kidney-friendly dialysis recipe is appropriate for kidney-friendly dialysis patients, but the above good kidney recipes are not suitable due to their low protein content. They aren't even good for kidney patients, because these foods, among other factors, stimulate inflammation. While they are not necessarily appropriate, they are also not suitable for kidneys - safe dialysis diet patients.

If you have kidney failure or are on dialysis, you must adhere to a kidney-friendly diet. If you have kidney disease or kidney dysfunction, you should incorporate this in your kidney diet guidelines, and the first step to a balanced kidney nutrition strategy is to supply your kitchen with the right foods.

If you don't practice the kidney diet, you should become a dietician. This cookbook contains information for those who follow a kidney or renal diet, as well as a list of kidney-friendly meals for dialysis and kidney patients. The handouts provide specifics about kidney function and recovery options, as well as patients who follow kidney / kidney diet guidelines. It's a safe place to start for people who have kidney disease, but it's also helpful for people who have kidney dysfunction or other illnesses.

BREAKFAST

1. Apple Sauce Cream Toast

Preparation Time: 5 minutes

Cooking Time: 10 Minutes

Servings: 1

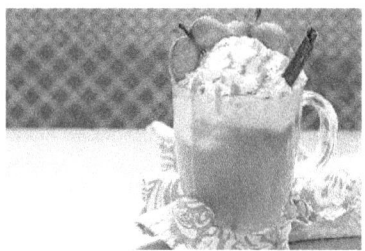

Ingredients:

- 2 tablespoons applesauce
- 2 slices of toast or white bread
- 1 egg white – uncooked, scrambled
- Cinnamon

Direction:

1. Whip the liquid uncooked egg white until foamy and take a skillet that doesn't stick. Heat the skillet then soak one side of the toast into the egg white whip.
2. Bake the toast on the side where the toast is soaked into the egg white and while you are doing so, soak another piece of toast into the egg white whip and as you are baking the second toast piece and applesauce on the

second piece and seal with the first piece of toast once the outside crust is well baked.

3. Sprinkle with cinnamon to taste and serve.

Nutrition: Potassium 294 mg Sodium 366 mg Phosphorus 158 mg Calories 256

2. Waffles

Preparation Time: 20 minutes

Cooking Time: 15 Minutes

Servings: 8

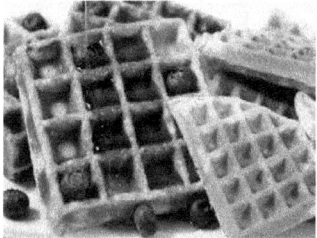

Ingredients:

- 1 and ½ teaspoons yeast for baking
- 8 tablespoons butter – unsalted
- 2 eggs
- 1 and ¾ cups of milk – 2% milkfat
- Sugar substitute to taste
- 1 teaspoon almond extract
- 2 cups flour – all-purpose

Direction:

1. Heat a saucepan and place the butter and milk in it. Wait for the butter to melt with occasional stirring. As you are waiting for the milk and butter mixture to cool off a bit so that the saucepan is warm to touch, you will take a bowl and whisk sugar substitute, yeast and flour. Once combined, you will add the warm milk and butter

mixture to the flour bowl and whisk some more until the mass is well combined.

2. Take another bowl and whisk the eggs with almond extract, adding the flour batter's whipped egg mixture. Stir in well to combine until you get a smooth, homogenous mass. The best option is to prepare the mixture a day ahead as you will need to keep the dough in the fridge for at least 12 hours before baking.

3. Once you are ready to bake your waffles, you will set the oven to 200 degrees F and keep the waffle bowl near so that the dough is kept warm. Prepare your waffle maker and start making waffles by pouring the dough.

Nutrition: Potassium 131 mg Sodium 208 mg Phosphorus 113 mg Calories 223

3. Egg Whites and Veggie Bake

Preparation Time: 20 minutes

Cooking Time: 50 Minutes

Servings: 4

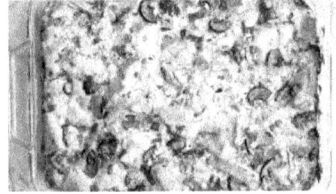

Ingredients:

- 1 cup broccoli florets
- 1 cup cauliflower florets
- 1 garlic clove - minced
- 6 egg whites – liquid, uncooked
- ½ cup bell pepper – diced
- 1 small onion – finely diced
- ½ cup low-sodium cheese

Direction:

1. Take care of the veggies, wash and dice the cauliflower, broccoli and onion. While you are sautéing onion with a tablespoon of olive oil, place broccoli and cauliflower in a bowl with a tablespoon water and place the bowl in the microwave.
2. Microwave florets for 5 minutes before taking the bowl out of the microwave. The onions should be ready

within 5 minutes, when you should add the minced garlic and peppers. Sauté for another 3 to 4 minutes.

3. Combine broccoli and cauliflower florets with garlic, peppers and onion and let the veggie mixture cool off a bit as you are whisking egg whites. Egg whites should be whisked until foamy. Whisk in the cheese with the egg whites then add the veggie mixture to your egg whites, stirring the ingredients to combine it into a homogenous mass.

4. Take a medium baking dish and pour in the mixture. Preheat the oven to 350 degrees F and place the baking dish into the oven, baking the egg white veggie bake for 20 minutes or until the mixture settles.

Nutrition: Potassium 163 mg Sodium 89 mg Phosphorus 105 mg Calories 258

4. Peach Berry Parfait

Preparation Time: 5 minutes

Cooking Time: 5 minutes

Servings: 2 servings

Ingredients:

- 1 cup plain, unsweetened yogurt, divided
- 1 teaspoon vanilla extract
- 1 small peach, diced
- ½ cup blueberries
- 2 tablespoons walnut pieces

Directions:

1. In a small bowl, combine the yogurt and vanilla.
2. Put 2 tablespoons of yogurt to each of 2 cups. Divide the diced peach and the blueberries between the cups, and top with the remaining yogurt.
3. Sprinkle each cup with 1 tablespoon of walnut pieces.

Nutrition: Calories: 191; Total Fat: 10g; Saturated Fat: 3g; Cholesterol: 15mg; Carbohydrates: 14g; Fiber: 14g; Protein: 12g; Phosphorus: 189mg; Potassium: 327mg; Sodium: 40mg

5. Open-Faced Bagel Breakfast Sandwich

Preparation Time: 5 minutes

Cooking Time: 5 minutes

Servings: 2 servings

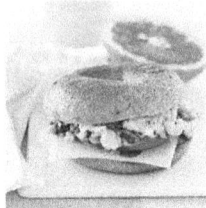

Ingredients:

- 1 multigrain bagel, halved
- 2 slices tomato
- 1 slice red onion
- Freshly ground black pepper
- 1 cup microgreens

Directions:

1. Lightly toast the bagel.
2. Place the bagel halves, top each half with 1 slice of tomato and a coupleof onion ringsn.
3. Season with the black pepper. Top each half with ½ cup of microgreens and serve.

Nutrition: Calories: 156; Total Fat: 6g; Saturated Fat: 3g; Cholesterol: 18mg; Carbohydrates: 22g; Fiber: 3g; Protein: 5g; Protein: 5g; Phosphorus: 98mg; Potassium: 163mg; Sodium: 195mg

6. Bulgur Bowl with Strawberries and Walnuts

Preparation Time: 10 minutes

Cooking Time: 15 minutes

Servings: 4 servings

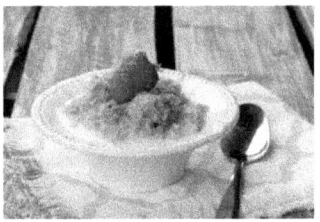

Ingredients:

- 1 cup bulgur
- 1 cup strawberries, sliced
- 4 tablespoons (¼ cup) homemade rice milk or unsweetened store-bought rice milk
- 4 teaspoons brown sugar
- 4 teaspoons extra-virgin olive oil
- 4 tablespoons (¼ cup) walnut pieces
- 4 tablespoons (¼ cup) cacao nibs (optional)

Directions:

1. In a small pot, combine the bulgur with 2 cups of water. Bring to a boil, lower the heat and let simmer, covered, for 12 to 15 minutes, until tender.
2. In each of four bowls, add a quarter of the bulgur and top with ¼ cup of strawberries, 1 tablespoon of rice

milk, 1 teaspoon of brown sugar, 1 teaspoon of olive oil, 1 tablespoon of walnut pieces, and 1 tablespoon of cacao nibs (if using).

Nutrition: Calories: 190; Total Fat: 9g; Saturated Fat: 1g; Cholesterol: 0mg; Carbohydrates: 26g; Fiber: 5g; Protein: 4g; Phosphorus: 66mg; Potassium: 153mg; Sodium: 13mg

7. Overnight oats three ways

Preparation Time: 5 minutes

Cooking Time: 5 minutes

Servings: 2 servings

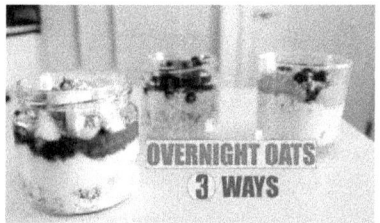

Ingredients:

- ¾ cup homemade rice milk or unsweetened store-bought rice milk
- ½ cup plain, unsweetened yogurt
- ½ cup rolled oats
- 1 tablespoon ground flaxseed
- 1 teaspoon vanilla extract
- 2 teaspoons honey

Directions:

1. In a medium bowl, mix the rice milk, yogurt, oats, flaxseed, vanilla, and honey.
2. Add the ingredients to make your preferred variation, and stir to blend.
3. Divide between two jars, cover, and refrigerate for at least 4 hours or overnight.

Nutrition: Calories: 196; Total Fat: 7g; Saturated Fat: 2g; Cholesterol: 7mg; Carbohydrates: 25g; Fiber: 3g; Protein: 8g; Phosphorus: 99mg; Potassium: 114mg; Sodium: 63mg

LUNCH

8. Chicken with Quinoa and Wild Rice

Preparation Time: 10 minutes

Cooking Time: 40 minutes

Servings: 4

Ingredients:

- ½ cup kale
- 1 cup red onion
- 10 garlic cloves
- 1 tablespoon olive oil
- 6 tablespoons lemon juice
- 1 tablespoon black pepper
- 1 cup quinoa, uncooked
- 1 cup white rice, uncooked
- 4 cups low-sodium chicken broth
- 2 pounds boneless, skinless chicken breast
- 5 tablespoons fresh basil

Directions:

1. Preheat oven to 375ºF.
2. Chop kale. Chop the red onion and garlic.
3. Add olive oil, 4 tablespoons of lemon juice, pepper, onion, garlic, quinoa and rice and chicken broth to a 9-inch x 13-inch baking pan. Mix ingredients together.
4. Add kale on top of rice mixture.

5. Add chicken breast on top of kale.
6. Cover with foil and bake for 45 minutes or until chicken is done and the majority of chicken broth has been absorbed.
7. Let sit for 5-10 minutes. While dish is cooling, chop fresh parsley and combine with remaining 2 tablespoon lemon juice. Sprinkle on top and enjoy!

Nutrition: Calories 146, Total Fat 2.7g, Saturated Fat 0.4g, Cholesterol 11mg, Sodium 40mg, Total Carbohydrate 21.8g, Dietary Fiber 2.4g, Total Sugar 1g, Protein 8.7g, Calcium 27mg, Iron 1mg, Potassium 270mg, Phosphorus 206 mg

9. Pineapple and Mint Lamb Chops

Preparation Time: 10 minutes

Cooking Time: 10 minutes

Servings: 4

Ingredients:

- 1/2 tablespoon olive oil
- 2 tablespoons pineapple juice
- ¼ tablespoon chopped fresh mint
- Salt and pepper to taste
- 4 lamb chops

Directions:

1. Stir together olive oil, pineapple juice, and mint in a small bowl. Season with salt and pepper to taste. Place lamb chops in a shallow dish, and brush with the olive oil mixture. Marinate in the refrigerator for 1 hour.
2. Preheat grill for high heat.
3. Lightly oil grill grate. Place lamb chops on grill, and discard marinade. Cook for 10 minutes, turning once, or to desired doneness.

Nutrition: Calories 137, Total Fat 6.4g, Saturated Fat 1.9g, Cholesterol 57mg, Sodium 49mg, Total Carbohydrate 0.8g, Dietary Fiber 0g, Total Sugar 0.7g,

10. Maple-Brined Pork Loin

Preparation Time: 15 minutes

Cooking Time: 60 minutes

Servings: 4

1-quart cold water

- 1/3 cup maple syrup
- 3 cloves garlic, crushed
- 3 tablespoons chopped fresh ginger
- 2 teaspoons dried rosemary
- 1 tablespoon cracked black pepper
- 1 boneless pork loin roast
- salt and freshly ground black pepper
- 1 tablespoon olive oil
- 2 tablespoons maple syrup
- 2 tablespoons Dijon mustard

Directions:

1. Mix water, salt, 1/3 cup maple syrup, garlic, ginger, rosemary, and black pepper, in a large bowl. Place pork loin in brine mixture and refrigerate for 8 to 10 hours.
2. Remove pork from brine, pat dry, and season all sides with salt and black pepper.
3. Preheat oven to 325 degrees F.
4. Heat olive oil in an oven-proof skillet over high heat. Cook pork, turning to brown each side, about 10 minutes' total.

5. Transfer skillet to the oven and roast until pork is browned, about 40 minutes.
6. Mix 2 tablespoons maple syrup and Dijon mustard together in a small bowl.
7. Remove pork roast from the oven and spread maple syrup mixture on all sides. Cook for an additional 15 minutes, until the pork is no longer pink in the center. An instant-read thermometer inserted into the center should read 145 degrees F.

Nutrition: Calories 158, Total Fat 5g, Saturated Fat 0.9g, Cholesterol 16mg, Sodium 106mg, Total Carbohydrate 23.1g, Dietary Fiber 1.5g, Total Sugar 15.9g,

DINNER

11. Falafel

Preparation Time: 10 minutes

Cooking time: 6 minutes

Servings: 4 servings

Ingredients:

- 1 cup chickpeas, soaked, cooked
- 1/3 cup white onion, diced
- 3 garlic cloves, chopped
- 3 tablespoons fresh parsley, chopped
- 1 tablespoon chickpea flour
- ½ teaspoon salt
- ½ teaspoon ground cumin
- ¾ teaspoon ground coriander
- ½ teaspoon chili flakes
- ½ teaspoon cayenne pepper
- ½ teaspoon ground cardamom
- 3 tablespoons olive oil

Directions:

1. Blend chickpeas, onion, garlic cloves, parsley, chickpea flour, salt, ground cumin, ground coriander, chili flakes, cayenne pepper ground cardamom.

2. When the chickpea mixture is homogenous and smooth transfer it in the mixing bowl.
3. Make the medium balls from the chickpea mixture.
4. Pour olive oil in the skillet and heat it.
5. Fry the chickpea balls for 2 minutes from each side over the medium heat.
6. The cooked falafel should have a light brown color.
7. Dry the falafel with a paper towel if needed.

Nutrition: calories 283, fat 13.7, fiber 9.2, carbs 32.6, protein 10.1

12. Israeli Pasta Salad

Preparation Time: 10 minutes

Cooking time: 15 minutes

Servings: 2 servings

Ingredients:

- 2 bell peppers, chopped
- 3 oz. Feta cheese, chopped
- 1 red onion, chopped
- 1 tomato, chopped
- 1 cucumber, chopped
- ½ cup elbow macaroni, dried
- 1 teaspoon dried oregano
- 1 tablespoon lemon juice
- 1 teaspoon olive oil
- 1 cup water for macaroni

Directions:

1. Pour water in the pan, add macaroni and boil them according to the
2. Directions of the manufacturer (appx. 15 minutes).
3. Then drain water and chill the macaroni little.
4. Meanwhile, in the salad bowl mix up together Feta cheese, bell peppers, onion, tomato, and cucumber.

5. Make the dressing for the salad: combine dried oregano, lemon juice, and olive oil.
6. Add cooked macaroni in the salad bowl and mix up well.
7. Drizzle the salad with dressing and shake gently.

Nutrition: calories 328, fat 14.8, fiber 5.6, carbs 40.3, protein 12.2

13. Artichoke Matzo Mina

Preparation Time: 10 minutes

Cooking time: 45 minutes

Servings: 6 servings

Ingredients:

- 4 sheets matzo
- ½ cup artichoke hearts
- 1 cup cream cheese
- ½ teaspoon salt
- 1 teaspoon ground black pepper
- 3 tablespoons fresh dill, chopped
- 3 eggs, beaten
- 1 teaspoon canola oil
- ½ cup cottage cheese

Directions:

1. In the bowl combine, salt, ground black pepper, dill, and cottage cheese.
2. Pour canola oil in the skillet, add artichoke hearts and roast them for 2-3 minutes over the medium heat. Stir them from time to time.
3. Then add roasted artichoke hearts in the cheese mixture.
4. Add eggs and stir until homogenous.

5. Place one sheet of matzo in the casserole mold.
6. Then spread it with cheese mixture generously.
7. Cover the cheese layer with the second sheet of matzo.
8. Repeat the steps till you use all ingredients.
9. Then preheat oven to 360F.
10. Bake matzo mina for 40 minutes.
11. Cut the cooked meal into the.

Nutrition: calories 272, fat 17.3, fiber 4.3, carbs 20.2, protein 11.8

14. Sautéed Chickpea and Lentil Mix

Preparation Time: 10 minutes

Cooking Time: 50 minutes

Servings: 4

Ingredients:

- 1 cup chickpeas, half-cooked
- 1 cup lentils
- 5 cups chicken stock
- ½ cup fresh cilantro, chopped
- 1 teaspoon salt
- ½ teaspoon chili flakes
- ¼ cup onion, diced
- 1 tablespoon tomato paste

Directions:

1. Place chickpeas in the pan. Add water, salt, and chili flakes.
2. Boil the chickpeas for 30 minutes over the medium heat.
3. Then add diced onion, lentils, and tomato paste. Stir well.
4. Close the lid and cook the mix for 15 minutes.
5. After this, add chopped cilantro, stir the meal well and cook it for 5 minutes more.
6. Let the cooked lunch chill little before serving.

Nutrition: Calories 370 Fat 4.3 Fiber 23.7 Carbs 61.6 Protein 23.2

MAIN DISHES

15. Quinoa & Veggie Croquettes

Preparation Time: 15 minutes

Cooking Time: 9 minutes

Servings: 12-15

Ingredients:

- 1 tbsp. essential olive oil
- ½ cup frozen peas, thawed
- 2 minced garlic cloves
- 1 cup cooked quinoa
- 2 large boiled carrots, peeled and mashed
- ¼ cup fresh cilantro leaves, chopped
- 2 teaspoons ground cumin
- 1 teaspoon garam masala
- ¼ teaspoon ground turmeric
- Salt, to taste
- Freshly ground black pepper, to taste
- Olive oil, for frying

Directions:

1. In a frying pan, warm oil on medium heat.
2. Add peas and garlic and sauté for about 1 minute.
3. Transfer the pea mixture into a large bowl.
4. Add the remainder ingredients and mix till well combined.

5. Make equal sized oblong shaped patties from your mixture.
6. In a huge skillet, heat oil on medium-high heat.
7. Add croquettes and fry for about 4 minutes per side.

Nutrition: Calories: 367 Fat: 6g Carbohydrates: 17g Fiber: 5g Protein: 22g

16. Salmon Burgers

Preparation Time: 15 minutes

Cooking Time: 8 minutes

Servings: 3

Ingredients:

- 1 (6-oz. can) skinless, boneless salmon, drained
- 1 celery rib, chopped
- ½ of a medium onion, chopped
- 2 large eggs
- 1 tablespoon plus 1 teaspoon coconut flour
- 1 tablespoon dried dill, crushed
- 1 teaspoon lemon
- Salt, to taste
- Freshly ground black pepper, to taste
- 3 tablespoons coconut oil

Directions:

1. In a substantial bowl, add salmon and which has a fork, break it into small pieces.
2. Add remaining ingredients excluding the for oil and mix till well combined.
3. Make 6 equal sized small patties from the mixture.
4. In a substantial skillet, melt coconut oil on medium-high heat.
5. Cook the patties for around 3-4 minutes per side.

Nutrition: Calories: 393 Fat: 12g Carbohydrates: 19g Fiber: 5g Protein: 24g

SNACKS

17. Parmesan quinoa with peas

Preparation time: 5 minutes

Cooking time: 20 minutes

Servings: 2

Ingredients

- Quinoa – .75 cup
- Water – 1.5 cups
- Green peas, thawed if frozen - .75 cup
- Black pepper, ground - .25 teaspoon
- Olive oil – 1.5 tablespoons
- Parmesan cheese, grated – 3 tablespoons

Directions

1. Place the uncooked quinoa in a fine metal sieve and rinse it well with water until there is no debris running off.

2. Place the quinoa and water in a metal saucepan and bring it to a boil over medium heat. Once it attains a boil, reduce it to a light simmer, cover the pot with a lid, and allow cooking until the water has all been absorbed. This should take fifteen to twenty minutes.

3. Allow the quinoa to sit with the lid on for five minutes after turning off the heat. Once it has set, use a fork to

fluff the quinoa and stir in the green peas, olive oil, and quinoa. Close the lid once again, allowing it to sit for five additional minutes to warm the peas and melt the cheese. Enjoy the quinoa while warm.

Nutrition: calories in individual servings: 386 protein grams: 13 phosphorus milligrams: 378 potassium milligrams: 465 sodium milligrams: 144 fat grams: 16 total carbohydrates grams: 47 net carbohydrates grams: 41

18. Mushroom orzo

Preparation time: 5 minutes

Cooking time: 20 minutes

Servings: 2

Ingredients

- Orzo - .75 cup
- Chicken broth, low-sodium – 1.25 cup
- Mushrooms, diced – 4 ounces
- Garlic, minced – 3 cloves
- Onion flakes, dehydrated – 1 tablespoon
- Olive oil – 1 tablespoon
- Sage, ground - .25 teaspoon

Directions

1. Place the diced mushrooms, olive oil, and garlic in a medium-sized metal saucepan and allow them to sauté over medium heat for five minutes. Add in the sage, onion flakes, orzo, and low-sodium chicken broth. Bring the mixture to a boil.
2. Reduce the heat of the skillet to a light simmer, cover the pot with a lid, and allow it to cook until all of the liquid has been absorbed about nine minutes. Fluff the orzo with a fork before serving.

Nutrition: calories in individual servings: 337 protein grams: 18 phosphorus milligrams: 63 potassium milligrams: 430

sodium milligrams: 43 fat grams: 8 total carbohydrates grams: 99 net carbohydrates grams: 95

19. Carrot and pineapple slaw

Preparation time: 5 minutes

Cooking time: 0 minute

Servings: 2

Ingredients

- Carrot matchsticks – 5 ounces
- Pineapple chunks, canned, liquid drained - .5 cup
- Grapes, sliced in half - .5 cup
- Pecan pieces - .25 cup
- Mayonnaise, low-sodium - .33 cup
- Lemon juice – 1 tablespoon

Directions

1. In a bowl, toss together the carrot matchsticks, drained pineapple chunks, sliced grapes, and pecan pieces. Stir in the low-sodium mayonnaise and lemon juice.
2. Cover the bowl with plastic wrap or a lid and then allow it to chill and marinate for at least an hour before serving. You can make this slaw up to a day in advance.

Nutrition: calories in individual servings: 264 protein grams: 2 phosphorus milligrams: 74 potassium milligrams: 423 sodium milligrams: 91 fat grams: 17 total carbohydrates grams: 29 net carbohydrates grams: 25

20. Sesame cucumber salad

Preparation time: 5 minutes

Cooking time: 0 minute

Servings: 2

Ingredients

- Cucumbers, thinly sliced – 1
- Sesame seeds - .5 teaspoon
- Rice wine vinegar – 1 tablespoon
- Sugar - .5 tablespoon
- Sesame seed oil – 1.5 tablespoons
- Red pepper flakes - .25 teaspoon

Directions

1. You want the cucumbers sliced as thinly as you can get them. While you can certainly do this with a knife, it is quicker and easier if you use a mandolin.
2. In a medium to a small bowl, whisk together the sesame seeds, rice wine vinegar, sugar, sesame seed oil, and red pepper flakes. Once well combined, add in the cucumbers and toss the vegetables in the vinaigrette. Serve immediately.

Nutrition: calories in individual servings: 92 protein grams: 1 phosphorus milligrams: 46 potassium milligrams: 250 sodium milligrams: 117 fat grams: 5

SOUP AND STEW

21. Stuffed bell pepper soup

Preparation time: 5 minutes

Cooking time: 20 minutes

Servings: 2

Ingredients

- Chicken broth, low-sodium – 2 cups
- Bell pepper, red, diced – 1
- Garlic, minced – 4 cloves
- Onion, diced - .5 cup
- Ground turkey – 4 ounces
- Olive oil – 2 teaspoons
- Italian seasoning – 1 teaspoon
- White rice, cooked – 1 cup
- Parsley, fresh, chopped – 1 tablespoon

Directions

1. Cook the ground turkey with the onion, olive oil, , and garlic until the turkey is fully cooked and no pink is remaining about five to seven minutes.

2. Add the black pepper, Italian seasoning, and bell pepper to the soup pot, allowing it to cook for three more minutes.

3. Into the pot, pour the low-sodium chicken broth, simmer the soup for fifteen minutes, until the bell peppers are tender. Stir in the cooked rice and parsley before serving.

Nutrition: calories in individual servings: 283 protein grams: 16 phosphorus milligrams: 183 potassium milligrams: 369 sodium milligrams: 85 fat grams: 9 total carbohydrates grams: 32 net carbohydrates grams: 30

22. Italian chicken stew

Preparation time: 20 minutes

Cooking time: 8 hours

Servings: 1

Ingredients

- 1/2-pound chicken breast, boneless, skinless, cubed
- 1/3 cup celery, chopped
- 1/2 cup carrot, chopped
- 1/2 cup onion, chopped
- 2 ounce any kind of mushrooms, sliced
- 1/4 teaspoon dill weed
- 1/2 teaspoon italian seasoning
- 1/4 teaspoon basil
- 1/4 teaspoon black pepper
- 1 tomato, diced – limit this

Directions

1. Place chicken breast cubes into the slow cooker.
2. Add in onion, carrot, italian seasoning, mushrooms, celery, basil, dill weed, and black pepper.
3. Cover and cook for 8 to 9 hours on low. Secure the lid.
4. After the 8-hour cooking cycle, turn off the heat. Adjust seasoning according to your preferred taste.
5. Serve warm.

Nutrition: protein: 29.9 g potassium: 89.6 mg sodium: 56.3 mg

23. Turkey pasta stew

Preparation time: 10 minutes

Cooking time: 8 hours

Servings: 1

Ingredients

- 1/2-pound ground turkey
- 1/2 cup carrots, sliced
- 1/2 fennel bulb, chopped
- 1/4 cup celery, sliced
- 1 cup chicken broth, low sodium
- 1/3 teaspoon garlic, minced
- 1/2 teaspoon oregano
- 1/2 teaspoon basil
- 1/2 cup shell pasta, uncooked
- 1 cup navy beans, unsalted, cooked

Directions

1. Cook turkey in a non-stick skillet set over medium heat until browned on all sides. Transfer to the slow cooker.
2. Add in garlic, carrots, chicken broth, navy beans, basil celery, pasta, oregano, and fennel. Stir well to combine.
3. Cover and cook for 8 to 9 hours on low. Secure the lid.

4. After the 8-hour cooking cycle, turn off the heat. Adjust seasoning according to your preferred taste. Serve warm.

Nutrition: protein: 18.8 g potassium: 84.6 mg sodium: 68.5 mg

24. One-pot chicken pie stew

Preparation time: 15 minutes

Cooking time: 1 hour 15 minutes

Servings: 8

Ingredients

- Fresh chicken breast (skinless and boneless) – 1½ pounds
- Low-sodium chicken stock – 2 cups
- Canola oil – ¼ cup
- Flour – ½ cup
- Fresh carrots (diced) – ½ cup
- Fresh onions (diced) – ½ cup
- Fresh celery (diced) – ¼ cup
- Black pepper – ½ teaspoon
- Italian seasoning (sodium-free) – 1 tablespoon
- Low-sodium better than bouillon® chicken base – 2 teaspoons
- Frozen sweet peas (thawed) – ½ cup
- Heavy cream – ½ cup
- Frozen piecrust (cooked, broken into bite-sized pieces) – 1
- Cheddar cheese (low-fat) – 1 cup

Directions

1. Start by pounding the chicken to tenderize it. Cut into small equal-sized cubes.
2. Place it over a medium-high flame. Add in the stock and the chicken. Cook for about 30 minutes.
3. Add in the flour and oil, while the chicken is cooking, mix well to combine.
4. Stir the flour and oil mixture into the broth mixture. Keep stirring until the chicken broth starts to thicken.
5. Reduce the flame to low and cook for another 15 minutes.
6. Now add in the carrots, celery, onions, italian seasoning, bouillon, and black pepper. Cook for another 15 minutes.
7. Add in the cream and peas after turning off the flame. Keep stirring to mix well.
8. Transfer into soup mugs and top with the cheese and broken pie crust pieces.

Nutrition: protein – 26 g   carbohydrates – 22 g fat – 21 g cholesterol – 82 mg sodium – 424 mg potassium – 209 mg phosphorus – 290 mg calcium – 88 mg fiber – 2 g

25. Spring Veggie Soup

Preparation Time: 20 minutes

Cooking Time: 45 minutes

Servings: 5

Ingredients:

- 2 tablespoons olive oil
- 1/2 cup onion, diced
- 1/2 cup mushrooms, sliced
- 1/8 cup celery, chopped
- 1 tomato, diced
- 1/2 cup carrots, diced
- 1 cup green beans, trimmed
- 1/2 cup frozen corn
- 1 teaspoon garlic powder
- 1 teaspoon dried oregano leaves
- 4 cups low-sodium vegetable broth

Directions:

1. In a pot, pour the olive oil and cook the onion and celery for 2 minutes.
2. Add the rest of the ingredients.
3. Bring to a boil.
4. Reduce heat and simmer for 45 minutes.

Nutrition: Calories: 136 Fat: 11g Carbohydrates: 17g Protein: 7g Sodium: 138mg Potassium: 527mg Phosphorus: 125mg

VEGETABLE

26. Crack Slaw

Preparation Time: 15 minutes

Cooking Time: 10 minutes

Servings: 6

Ingredients:

- 1 cup cauliflower rice
- 1 tablespoon sriracha
- 1 teaspoon tahini paste
- 1 teaspoon sesame seeds
- 1 tablespoon lemon juice
- 1 teaspoon olive oil
- 1 teaspoon butter
- ½ teaspoon salt
- 2 cups coleslaw

Directions:

1. Toss the butter in the skillet and melt it.
2. Add cauliflower rice and sprinkle it with sriracha and tahini paste.
3. Mix up the vegetables and cook them for 10 minutes over the medium heat. Stir them from time to time.
4. When the cauliflower is cooked, transfer it into the big plate.
5. Add coleslaw and stir gently.

6. Then sprinkle the salad with sesame seeds, lemon juice, olive oil, and salt.
7. Mix up well.

Nutrition: Calories 76, Fat 5.8, Fiber 0.6, Carbs 6, Protein 1.1

27. Vegan Chili

Preparation Time: 10 minutes

Cooking Time: 20 minutes

Servings: 4

Ingredients:

- 1 cup cremini mushrooms, chopped
- 1 zucchini, chopped
- 1 bell pepper, diced
- 1/3 cup crushed Red bell peppers
- 1 oz. celery stalk, chopped
- 1 teaspoon chili powder
- 1 teaspoon salt
- ½ teaspoon chili flakes
- ½ cup of water
- 1 tablespoon olive oil
- ½ teaspoon diced garlic
- ½ teaspoon ground black pepper
- 1 teaspoon of cocoa powder
- 2 oz. Cheddar cheese, grated

Directions:

1. Pour olive oil in the pan and preheat it.
2. Add chopped mushrooms and roast them for 5 minutes. Stir them from time to time.
3. After this, add chopped zucchini and bell pepper.
4. Sprinkle the vegetables with the chili powder, salt, chili flakes, diced garlic, and ground black pepper.
5. Stir the vegetables and cook them for 5 minutes more.

6. After this, add crushed Red bell peppers. Mix up well.
7. Bring the mixture to boil and add water and cocoa powder.
8. Then add celery stalk.
9. Mix up the chili well and close the lid.
10. Cook the chili for 10 minutes over the medium-low heat.
11. Then transfer the cooked vegan chili in the bowls and top with the grated cheese.

Nutrition: Calories 123, Fat 8.6, Fiber 2.3, Carbs 7.6, Protein 5.6

28. Chow Mein

Preparation Time: 10 minutes

Cooking Time: 10 minutes

Servings: 6

Ingredients:

- 7 oz. kelp noodles
- 5 oz. broccoli florets
- 1 tablespoon tahini sauce
- ¼ teaspoon minced ginger
- 1 teaspoon Sriracha
- ½ teaspoon garlic powder
- 1 cup of water

Directions:

1. Boil water in a sauce pan.
2. Add broccoli and boil for 4 minutes over the high heat.
3. Then drain water into the bowl and chill it tills the room temperature.
4. Soak the kelp noodles in the "broccoli water".
5. Meanwhile, place tahini sauce, sriracha, minced ginger, and garlic in the saucepan.
6. Bring the mixture to boil. Add oil if needed.
7. Then add broccoli and soaked noodles.
8. Add 3 tablespoons of "broccoli water".
9. Mix up the noodles and bring to boil.
10. Switch off the heat and transfer chow Mein in the serving bowls.

Nutrition: Calories 18, Fat 0.8, Fiber 0.7, Carbs 2.8, Protein 0.9

29. Mushroom Tacos

Preparation Time: 10 minutes

Cooking Time: 15 minutes

Servings: 6

Ingredients:

- 6 collard greens leave
- 2 cups mushrooms, chopped
- 1 white onion, diced
- 1 tablespoon Taco seasoning
- 1 tablespoon coconut oil
- ½ teaspoon salt
- ¼ cup fresh parsley
- 1 tablespoon mayonnaise

Directions:

1. Put the coconut oil in the skillet and melt it.
2. Add chopped mushrooms and diced onion. Mix up the ingredients.
3. Close the lid and cook them for 10 minutes.
4. After this, sprinkle the vegetables with Taco seasoning, salt, and add fresh parsley.
5. Mix up the mixture and cook for 5 minutes more.
6. Then add mayonnaise and stir well.
7. Chill the mushroom mixture little.
8. Fill the collard green leaves with the mushroom mixture and fold up them.

Nutrition: Calories 52, Fat 3.3, Fiber 1.2, Carbs 5.1, Protein 1.4

SIDE DISHES

30. Chicken and Mandarin Salad

Preparation time: 40 minutes

Cooking time: 30 minutes

Servings: 3

Ingredients:

- 1 ½ - cup Chicken
- ½ - cup Celery
- ½ - cup Green pepper
- ¼ - cup Onion, finely sliced
- ¼ - cup Light mayonnaise
- ½ - tsp. freshly ground pepper

Directions:

1. Hurl chicken, celery, green pepper and onion to blend. Include mayo and pepper. Blend delicately and serve.

Nutrition: Calories 375, Fat 15, Fiber 2, Carbs 14, Protein 28

SALAD

31. Italian Cucumber Salad

Preparation Time: 5 minutes

Cooking Time: 0 minutes

Servings: 2

Ingredients:

- 1/4 cup rice vinegar
- 1/8 teaspoon stevia
- 1/2 teaspoon olive oil
- 1/8 teaspoon black pepper
- 1/2 cucumber, sliced
- 1 cup carrots, sliced
- 2 tablespoons green onion, sliced
- 2 tablespoons red bell pepper, sliced
- 1/2 teaspoon Italian seasoning blend

Direction:

1. Put all the salad ingredients into a suitable salad bowl.
2. Toss them well and refrigerate for 1 hour.
3. Serve.

Nutrition: Calories 112 Total Fat 1.6g Cholesterol 0mg Sodium 43mg Protein 2.3g Phosphorous 198mg Potassium 529mg

32. Grapes Jicama Salad

Preparation Time: 5 minutes

Cooking Time: 0 minutes

Servings: 2

Ingredients:

- 1 jicama, peeled and sliced
- 1 carrot, sliced
- 1/2 medium red onion, sliced
- 1 ¼ cup seedless grapes
- 1/3 cup fresh basil leaves
- 1 tablespoon apple cider vinegar
- 1 ½ tablespoon lemon juice
- 1 ½ tablespoon lime juice

Direction:

1. Put all the salad ingredients into a suitable salad bowl.
2. Toss them well and refrigerate for 1 hour.
3. Serve.

Nutrition: Calories 203 Total Fat 0.7g Sodium 44mg Protein 3.7g Calcium 79mg Phosphorous 141mg Potassium 429mg

FISH & SEAFOOD

33. Spanish Tuna

Preparation Time: 20 minutes

Cooking Time: 15 minutes

Servings: 4

Ingredients:

- 1 tablespoon olive oil
- 1/4 cup finely chopped onion
- 2 tablespoons chopped fresh garlic
- 1/4 cup basil chopped
- 1 dash black pepper
- 1 dash cayenne pepper
- 1 dash paprika
- 6 (4 ounce) fillets tuna fillets

Directions:

1. Heat olive oil in a large skillet over medium heat.
2. Cook and stir onions and garlic until onions are slightly tender, careful not to burn the garlic.
3. Season with black pepper, cayenne pepper, basil, and paprika.

4. Cook fillets in sauce over medium heat for 5 to 8 minutes, or until easily flaked with a fork. Serve immediately.

Nutrition: Calories 130, Total Fat 4.6g, Saturated Fat 0.5g, Cholesterol 55mg, Sodium 71mg, Total Carbohydrate 2.2g, Dietary Fiber 0.3g, Total Sugar 0.4g, Protein 20.4g, Calcium 10mg, Iron 0mg, Potassium 31mg, Phosphorus 46 mg

34. Fish with Vegetables

Preparation Time: 30 minutes

Cooking Time: 60 minutes

Servings: 4

Ingredients:

- 1 egg white, beaten
- ¼ cup all-purpose flour
- Black pepper to taste
- 1-pound firm salmon fillets, cut into 1 1/2-inch pieces
- ½ cup olive oil, divided
- 1 onion, cut in half and thinly sliced
- 1 carrot, peeled and coarsely grated
- ½ large turnips, peeled and coarsely grated
- 1/2 leek coarsely grated
- 1 cup water

Directions:

1. Place egg white and flour in 2 shallow bowls. Season egg white with pepper. Dip fish pieces first in the beaten egg, then dredge in the flour.
2. Heat 1/4 cup olive oil in a deep skillet over medium heat until hot. Add fish in batches and fry on both sides until golden, 5 to 8 minutes per batch. Remove fish from skillet and set aside.

3. Heat remaining 1/4 cup oil in a separate skillet and cook onions until soft and translucent, about 5 minutes. Add carrots, turnips, and leek; mix well. Add water and season with pepper. Cover and simmer on low heat until vegetables are soft, about 30 minutes. Check and add more water if mixture becomes too dry.

4. Layer vegetables and fried fish in a 10-inch round serving dish, starting and ending with vegetables.

Nutrition: Calories 358, Total Fat 30.1g, Saturated Fat 6g, Cholesterol 57mg, Sodium 45mg, Total Carbohydrate 14.7g, Dietary Fiber 2.2g, Total Sugar 3.3g, Protein 8.2g, Calcium 38mg, Iron 1mg, Potassium 281mg, Phosphorus 161 mg

35. Creamy Crab over Salmon

Preparation Time: 10 minutes

Cooking Time: 15 minutes

Servings: 4

Ingredients:

- 1/4 cup olive oil, divided
- 2 (4 ounce) fillets salmon
- 1 teaspoon dried oregano
- 1 pinch ground white pepper
- 1 3/4 cups soy almond milk
- 4 ounces' fresh crabmeat
- 1 teaspoon lemon juice

Directions:

1. Heat a small amount of the olive oil in a non-stick skillet over medium heat. Season salmon with oregano, and white pepper; cook in skillet until the flesh flakes easily with a fork, 7 to 10 minutes per side.

2. While fish cooks, whisk remaining olive oil, soy almond milk, together in a saucepan over medium-low heat; cook, stirring regularly, until it thickens, 3 to 5 minutes. Remove saucepan from heat and stir crabmeat into the sauce.

3. Transfer cooked cod to plates and spoon sauce over the fish.

Nutrition: Calories 258, Total Fat 16.5g, Saturated Fat 2.5g, Cholesterol 40mg, Sodium 395mg, Total Carbohydrate 11.4g, Dietary Fiber 1g, Total Sugar 6.1g, Protein 17.3g, Calcium 37mg, Iron 1mg, Potassium 160mg, Potassium 120mg

36. Curried fish cakes

Preparation time: 10 minutes

Cooking time: 18 minutes

Servings: 4

Ingredients

- ¾ pound Atlantic cod, cubed
- 1 apple, peeled and cubed
- 1 tablespoon yellow curry paste
- 2 tablespoons cornstarch
- 1 tablespoon peeled grated ginger root
- 1 large egg
- 1 tablespoon freshly squeezed lemon juice
- 1/8 teaspoon freshly ground black pepper
- ½ cup crushed puffed rice cereal
- 1 tablespoon olive oil

Directions

1. Put the cod, apple, curry, cornstarch, ginger, egg, lemon juice, and pepper in a blender or food processor and process until finely chopped. Avoid over-processing, or the mixture will become mushy.
2. Place the rice cereal on a shallow plate.
3. Form the mixture into 8 patties.
4. Dredge the patties in the rice cereal to coat.

5. Cook patties for 3 to 5 minutes per side, turning once until a meat thermometer registers 160°f.
6. Serve.

Nutrition: per serving: calories: 188; total fat: 6g; saturated fat: 1g; sodium: 150mg; potassium: 292mg; phosphorus: 150mg; carbohydrates: 12g; fiber: 1g; protein: 21g; sugar: 5g

37. Baked sole with caramelized onion

Preparation time: 10 minutes

Cooking time: 20 minutes

Servings: 4

Ingredients

- 1 cup finely chopped onion
- ½ cup low-sodium vegetable broth
- 1 yellow summer squash, sliced
- 2 cups frozen broccoli florets
- 4 (3-ounce) fillets of sole
- Pinch salt
- 2 tablespoons olive oil
- Pinch baking soda
- 1 teaspoon dried basil leaves

Directions

1. Preheat the oven to 425°f.
2. Add the onions. Cook for 1 minute; then, stirring constantly, cook for another 4 minutes.
3. Remove the onions from the heat.
4. Pour the broth into a baking sheet with a lip and arrange the squash and broccoli on the sheet in a single layer. Top the vegetables with the fish. Sprinkle the fish with the salt and drizzle everything with the olive oil.

5. Bake the fish and the vegetables for 10 minutes.
6. While the fish is baking, return the skillet with the onions to medium-high heat and stir in a pinch of baking soda.
7. Transfer the onions to a plate.
8. Top the fish evenly with the onions. Sprinkle with the basil.
9. Return the fish to the oven, after this bake it 8 to10 minutes serve the fish on the vegetables.

Nutrition: per serving: calories: 202; total fat: 11g; saturated fat: 3g; sodium: 320mg; potassium: 537; phosphorus: 331mg; carbohydrates: 10g; fiber: 3g; protein: 16g; sugar: 4g

POULTRY RECIPES

38. Grilled Chicken with Pineapple & Veggies

Preparation Time: 20 or so minutes

Cooking Time: 22 minutes

Servings: 4

Ingredients:

- For Sauce:
- 1 garlic oil, minced
- ¾ teaspoon fresh ginger, minced
- ½ cup coconut aminos
- ¼ cup fresh pineapple juice
- 2 tablespoons freshly squeezed lemon juice
- 2 tablespoons balsamic vinegar
- ¼ teaspoon red pepper flakes, crushed
- Salt
- ground black pepper
- For Grilling:
- 4 skinless, boneless chicken breasts
- 1 pineapple, peeled and sliced
- 1 bell pepper, seeded and cubed
- 1 zucchini, sliced
- 1red onion, sliced

Directions:

1. For sauce in a pan, mix all ingredients on medium-high heat. Bring to a boil reducing the heat to medium-low. Cook approximately 5-6 minutes.
2. Remove, then keep aside to cool down slightly. Coat the chicken breasts about ¼ from the sauce. Keep aside for approximately half an hour.
3. Preheat the grill to medium-high heat. Grease the grill grate. Grill the chicken pieces for around 5-8 minutes per side.
4. Now, squeeze pineapple and vegetables on the grill grate. Grill the pineapple within 3 minutes per side. Grill the vegetables for approximately 4-5 minutes, stirring once inside the middle way.
5. Cut the chicken breasts into desired size slices, divide the chicken, pineapple, and vegetables into serving plates. Serve alongside the remaining sauce.

Nutrition: Calories: 435 Fat: 12g Carbohydrates: 25g Protein: 38g Phosphorus 184 mg Potassium 334.4 mg Sodium 755.6 mg

39. Ground Turkey with Veggies

Preparation Time: 15 minutes

Cooking Time: 12 minutes

Servings: 4

Ingredients:

- 1 tablespoon sesame oil
- 1 tablespoon coconut oil
- 1-pound lean ground turkey
- 2 tablespoons fresh ginger, minced
- 2 minced garlic cloves
- 1 (16-ounce) bag vegetable mix (broccoli, carrot, cabbage, kale, and Brussels sprouts)
- ¼ cup coconut aminos
- 2 tablespoons balsamic vinegar

Directions:

1. In a big skillet, heat both oils on medium-high heat. Add turkey, ginger, and garlic and cook approximately 5-6 minutes. Add vegetable mix and cook about 4-5 minutes. Stir in coconut aminos and vinegar and cook for about 1 minute. Serve hot.

Nutrition: Calories: 234 Fat: 9g Carbohydrates: 9g Protein: 29g Phosphorus 14 mg Potassium 92.2 mg Sodium 114.9 mg

40. Ground Turkey with Asparagus

Preparation Time: 15 minutes

Cooking Time: 15 minutes

Servings: 8

Ingredients:

- 1¾ pound lean ground turkey
- 2 tablespoons sesame oil
- 1 medium onion, chopped
- 1 cup celery, chopped
- 6 garlic cloves, minced
- 2 cups asparagus, cut into 1-inch pieces
- 1/3 cup coconut aminos
- 2½ teaspoons ginger powder
- 2 tablespoons organic coconut crystals
- 1 tablespoon arrowroot starch
- 1 tablespoon cold water
- ¼ teaspoon red pepper flakes, crushed

Directions:

1. Heat a substantial nonstick skillet on medium-high heat. Add turkey and cook for approximately 5-7 minutes or till browned. With a slotted spoon, transfer the turkey inside a bowl and discard the grease from the skillet.
2. Heat-up oil on medium heat in the same skillet. Add onion, celery, and garlic and sauté for about 5 minutes. Add asparagus and cooked turkey, minimizing the temperature to medium-low.

3. Meanwhile, inside a pan, mix coconut aminos, ginger powder, and coconut crystals n medium heat and convey some boil.
4. Mix arrowroot starch and water in a smaller bowl. Slowly add arrowroot mixture, stirring continuously. Cook approximately 2-3 minutes.
5. Add the sauce in the skillet with turkey mixture and stir to blend. Stir in red pepper flakes and cook for approximately 2-3 minutes. Serve hot.

Nutrition: Calories: 309 Fat: 20g Carbohydrates: 19g Protein: 28g Potassium 196.4 mg Sodium 77.8 mg Phosphorus 0 mg

41. Ground Turkey with Peas & Potato

Preparation Time: 15 minutes

Cooking Time: 35 minutes

Servings: 4

Ingredients:

- 3-4 tablespoons coconut oil
- 1-pound lean ground turkey
- 1-2 fresh red chilis, chopped
- 1 onion, chopped
- Salt, to taste
- 2 minced garlic cloves
- 1 (1-inch) piece fresh ginger, grated finely
- 1 tablespoon curry powder
- 1 teaspoon ground coriander
- 1 teaspoon ground cumin
- 1 teaspoon ground turmeric
- 2 large Yukon gold carrots, cubed into 1-inch size
- ½ cup of water
- 1 cup fresh peas, shelled
- 2-4 plum Red bell peppers, chopped
- ½ cup fresh cilantro, chopped

Directions:

1. In a substantial pan, heat oil on medium-high heat. Add turkey and cook for about 4-5 minutes. Add chilis and onion and cook for about 4-5 minutes.

2. Add garlic and ginger and cook approximately 1-2 minutes. Stir in spices, carrots, and water and convey to your boil
3. Reduce the warmth to medium-low. Simmer covered around 15-20 or so minutes. Add peas and Red bell peppers and cook for about 2-3 minutes. Serve using the garnishing of cilantro.

Nutrition: Calories: 452 Fat: 14g Carbohydrates: 24g Fiber: 13g Protein: 36g Phosphorus 38 mg Potassium 99.5 mg Sodium 373.4 mg

MEAT RECIPES

42. Beef Brochettes

Preparation Time: 20 minutes

Cooking Time: 1 hour

Servings: 1

Ingredients

- 1 1/2 cups pineapple chunks
- 1 sliced large onion
- 2 pounds thick steak
- 1 sliced medium bell pepper
- 1 bay leaf
- 1/4 cup vegetable oil
- 1/2 cup lemon juice
- 2 crushed garlic cloves

Directions

1. Cut beef cubes and place in a plastic bag
2. Combine marinade ingredients in small bowl
3. Mix and pour over beef cubes
4. Seal the bag and refrigerate for 3 to 5 hours
5. Divide ingredients onion, beef cube, green pepper, pineapple

6. Grill about 9 minutes each side

Nutrition: Calories 304 Protein 35 g Fat 15 g Carbs 11 g Phosphorus 264 mg Potassium (K) 388 mg Sodium (Na) 70 mg

43. Country Fried Steak

Preparation Time: 10 minutes

Cooking Time: 1 hour and 40 minutes

Servings: 3

Ingredients

- 1 large onion
- 1/2 cup flour
- 3 tablespoons. vegetable oil
- 1/4 teaspoon pepper
- 11/2 pounds round steak
- 1/2 teaspoon paprika

Directions

1. Trim excess fat from steak
2. Cut into small pieces
3. Combine flour, paprika and pepper and mix together
4. Preheat skillet with oil
5. Cook steak on both sides
6. When the color of steak is brown remove to a platter
7. Add water (150 ml) and stir around the skillet
8. Return browned steak to skillet, if necessary, add water again so that bottom side of steak does not stick

Nutrition: Calories 248 Protein 30 g Fat 10 g Carbs 5 g Phosphorus 190 mg Potassium (K) 338 mg Sodium (Na) 60 mg

BROTHS, CONDIMENT AND SEASONING

44. Salsa Verde

Preparation Time: 20 minutes

Cooking Time: 15 minutes

Servings: 2 cups

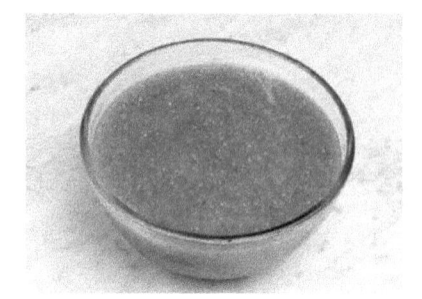

Ingredients:

- 2 cups halved tomatillos or 1 can tomatillos, drained
- 3 scallions, chopped
- 1 jalapeño pepper, chopped
- 2 tablespoons extra-virgin olive oil
- 1/3 cup cilantro leaves
- 2 tablespoons freshly squeezed lime juice
- 1/8 teaspoon salt

Directions:

1. Preheat the oven to 400°F. Mix the tomatillos, scallions, and jalapeño pepper on a rimmed baking sheet.

2. Drizzle using the olive oil, then toss to coat. Roast the vegetables for 12 to 17 minutes or until the tomatillos are soft and light golden brown around the edges.
3. Blend the roasted vegetables with the cilantro, lime juice, and salt in a blender or food processor. Blend until smooth. Store.

Nutrition: Calories: 22 Fat: 2g Sodium: 20mg Phosphorus: 8mg Potassium: 55mg Carbohydrates: 1g Protein: 0g

45. Grape Salsa

Preparation Time: 15 minutes

Cooking Time: 0 minutes

Servings: 2 cups

Ingredients:

- 1 cup coarsely chopped red grapes
- 1 cup coarsely chopped green grapes
- ½ cup chopped red onion
- 2 tablespoons freshly squeezed lime juice
- 1 tablespoon honey
- 1/8 teaspoon salt
- ¼ teaspoon freshly ground black pepper

Directions:

1. Mix the grapes, onion, lime juice, honey, salt, and pepper in a medium bowl. Chill within 1 to 2 hours before serving or serve immediately.

Nutrition: Calories: 51 Fat: 0g Sodium: 53mg Phosphorus: 14mg Potassium: 121mg Carbohydrates: 14g Protein: 1g

46. Apple and Brown Sugar Chutney

Preparation Time: 15 minutes

Cooking Time: 60 minutes

Servings: 2 cups

Ingredients:

- 3 Granny Smith apples, peeled and chopped
- 1 onion, chopped
- 1 cup of water
- 1/3 cup brown sugar
- 2 teaspoons curry powder
- 1/8 teaspoon salt
- 1/8 teaspoon freshly ground black pepper

Directions:

1. In a medium saucepan, combine the apples, onion, water, brown sugar, curry powder, and salt, plus pepper, then boil over medium-high heat.
2. Adjust the heat to low, then simmer, occasionally stirring, for 45 to 55 minutes. Cool, then decant into jars or containers. Store.

Nutrition: Calories: 27 Fat: 0g Sodium: 11mg Phosphorus: 6mg Potassium: 48mg Carbohydrates: 7g Protein: 0g

DRINKS AND SMOOTHIES

47. Honey Cinnamon Latte

Preparation Time: 5 minutes

Cooking Time: 5 minutes

Servings: 2

Ingredients:

- 1-½ cups of organic, unsweetened almond milk
- 1 scoop of organic vanilla protein powder
- 1 teaspoon of organic cinnamon
- ½ teaspoon of pure, local honey
- 1-2 shots of espresso

Directions:

1. Heat almond milk in the microwave until hot to the touch.
2. Add honey and stir until completely melted.
3. Using a whisk, add cinnamon, and protein powder and thoroughly combine.
4. Pour into a manual milk and froth concoction until foamy and creamy.
5. Pour espresso shots into a mug and add in milk mixture.

Nutrition: Calories: 115 Fat: 3g Carbs: 26g Protein: 3g Sodium: 125mg Potassium: 10.9mg Phosphorus: 0.1mg

48. Cinnamon Smoothie

Preparation Time: 5 minutes

Cooking Time: 5 minutes

Servings: 2

Ingredients:

- 150g plain or Greek yogurt
- 300ml milk
- 2 tbsp smooth peanut butter
- 1/4 tsp Schwartz Ground Cinnamon

Directions:

1. Add all the ingredients to a blender and blitz until smooth.
2. Serve immediately.

Nutrition: Calories: 88 Fat: 4.3g Carbs: 3g Protein: 8g Sodium: 187mg Potassium: 241mg Phosphorus: 20mg

DESSERT

49. Smooth Coffee Mousse

Preparation Time: 5 minutes

Cooking Time: 5 minutes

Servings: 8

Ingredients:

- 1 cup heavy whipping cream
- 1/2 cup unsweetened almond milk
- 4 tbsp brewed coffee
- 15 oz cream cheese, softened
- 15 drops liquid stevia
- 1 tsp vanilla

Directions:

1. Add coffee and cream cheese in a blender and blend until smooth.
2. Add stevia, vanilla, and almond milk and blend until smooth.
3. Add heavy cream and blend until thickened.
4. Pour into the serving bowls and place in refrigerator 1-2 hours.
5. Serve and enjoy.

Nutrition: Calories 241 Fat 24.3 g Carbohydrates 2 g Sugar 0.2 g Protein 4.4 g Cholesterol 79 mg Phosphorus: 80mg Potassium: 117mg Sodium: 75mg

50. Almond Bites

Preparation Time: 10 minutes

Cooking Time: 10 minutes

Servings: 12

Ingredients:

- 1/2 cup almond meal
- 2 tbsp coconut butter
- 4 dates, pitted and chopped
- 1/4 cup unsweetened chocolate chips
- 1 1/2 tsp vanilla

Directions:

1. Add dates in the food processor and process for 30 seconds.
2. Add remaining ingredients except chocolate chips and process until combined.
3. Add chocolate chips and process for 15 seconds.
4. Make small balls from mixture and place on a baking tray.
5. Place in refrigerator for 1-2 hours.
6. Serve and enjoy

Nutrition: Calories 53 Fat 3.8 g Carbohydrates 4.2 g Sugar 2.2 g Protein 1.1 g Cholesterol 1 mg Phosphorus: 110mg Potassium: 117mg Sodium: 75mg

51. Bacon Bell Peppers

Preapration Time:10 Minutes

Cooking Time: 5 Minutes

Servings: 16

Ingredients:

1 pack bacon slices

12 bell peppers, sliced in half

8 oz. cream cheese

Directions:

1. Stuff bell pepper halves with cream cheese.
2. Wrap with bacon slices.
3. Preheat Power XL Grill to 500 degrees F.
4. Add bell peppers to the grill.
5. Grill for 3 to 5 minutes.

Nutrition: Calories - 482 Fat – 42g Carbohydrates – 14g Fiber – 5g Protein – 28g

52. Corn & Carrot Fritters

Preapration Time:8 to 10 Minutes

Cooking Time: 12 Minutes

Servings: 4 to 5

Ingredients:

- 4 ounces canned sweet corn kernels, drained
- 1 teaspoon sea salt flakes
- 1 tablespoon cilantro, chopped
- 1 carrot, grated
- 1 yellow onion, finely chopped
- 1 medium-sized egg, whisked
- 1/4 cup of self-rising flour
- 1/3 teaspoon baking powder
- 2 tablespoons milk
- 1 cup Parmesan cheese, grated
- 1/3 teaspoon brown sugar

Directions:

1. Place your air fryer on a flat kitchen surface; plug it and turn it on. Set temperature to 350 degrees F and let it preheat for 4-5 minutes.
2. Press the carrot in the colander to remove excess liquid. Arrange the carrot between several sheets of kitchen towels and pat it dry.
3. Then, mix the carrots with the remaining Ingredients:in a big bowl. Make small balls from the mixture.

4. Gently flatten them with your hand. Spitz the balls with a nonstick cooking oil.
5. Add the in balls the basket.
6. Push the air-frying basket in the air fryer. Cook for 8-10 minutes.
7. Slide out the basket; serve warm!

Nutrition: Calories - 274 Fat – 8.3g Carbohydrates – 38.8g Fiber – 2.3g Protein – 15.6g

53. Butter Baked Nuts

Preapration Time:10 Minutes

Cooking Time: 15 Minutes

Servings: 4

Ingredients:

- 1 cup raw almonds or pistachios
- 1 cup raw peanuts
- 1 tablespoon butter, melted
- ½ cup raw cashew nuts
- Salt to taste

Directions:

1. Take Power XL multi-cooker, arrange it over a cooking platform, and open the top lid.
2. In the pot, arrange a reversible rack and place the Crisping Basket over the rack.
3. In the basket, add the nuts.
4. Seal the multi-cooker by locking it with the crisping lid; ensure to keep the pressure release valve locked/sealed.
5. Select the "AIR CRISP" mode and adjust the 350°F temperature level. Then, set Timer to 10 minutes and press "STOP/START"; it will start the cooking process by building up inside pressure.
6. When the Timer goes off, quick release pressure by adjusting the pressure valve to the VENT.
7. After pressure gets released, open the pressure lid.

8. Add the butter on top and season with some salt; shake well.
9. Seal the multi-cooker by locking it with the crisping lid; ensure to keep the pressure release valve locked/sealed.
10. Select "BAKE/ROAST" mode and adjust the 350°F temperature level. Then, set Timer to 5 minutes and press "STOP/START"; it will start the cooking process by building up inside pressure.
11. When the Timer goes off, quick release pressure by adjusting the pressure valve to the VENT. After pressure gets released, open the pressure lid.
12. Serve warm and enjoy!

Nutrition: Calories: 192 Fat: 16g Saturated Fat: 2g Trans Fat: 0g Carbohydrates: 6.5g Fiber: 3g Sodium: 64mg Protein: 7.5g

54. Eggs Spinach Side

Preapration Time:5 Minutes

Cooking Time: 12 Minutes

Servings: 2 to 3

Ingredients:

- 1 medium-sized tomato, chopped
- 1 teaspoon lemon juice
- 1/2 teaspoon coarse salt
- 2 tablespoons olive oil
- 4 eggs, whisked
- 5 ounces spinach, chopped
- 1/2 teaspoon black pepper
- 1/2 cup basil, roughly chopped

Directions:

1. Place your air fryer on a flat kitchen surface; plug it and turn it on. Set temperature to 280 degrees F and let it preheat for 4-5 minutes.
2. Take out the air-frying basket and gently coat it using the olive oil.
3. In a bowl of medium size, thoroughly mix the Ingredients:except for the basil leaves.
4. Add the mixture to the basket. Push the air-frying basket in the air fryer. Cook for 10-12 minutes.
5. Slide out the basket; top with basil and serve warm with sour cream!

Nutrition: Calories – 272 Fat, – 23g Carbohydrates – 5.4g Fiber – 2g Protein – 13.2g

55. Squash and Cumin Chili

Preapration Time:10 Minutes

Cooking Time: 16 Minutes

Servings: 4

Ingredients:

- One medium butternut squash
- One teaspoon cumin seed
- One large pinch of chili flakes
- One tablespoon olive oil
- One and ½ ounces pine nuts
- One small bunch of fresh coriander, chopped

Directions:

1. Take the squash and slice it
2. Remove seeds and cut into smaller chunks
3. Take a bowl and add chunked squash, spice, and oil
4. Mix well
5. Pre-heat your Fryer to 360 degrees F and add the squash to the cooking basket
6. Roast for 20 minutes. Ensure to shake the basket from Time to Time to avoid burning
7. Take a pan and place it over medium heat, add pine nuts to the pan, and dry toast for 2 minutes
8. Sprinkle nuts on top of the squash and serve
9. Enjoy!

Nutrition: Calories: 414 Fat: 15g Carbohydrates: 10g Protein: 16g

56. Fried Up Avocados

Preapration Time: 10 Minutes

Cooking Time: 20 Minutes

Servings: 6

Ingredients:

- ½ cup almond meal
- ½ teaspoon salt
- 1 Hass avocado, peeled, pitted, and sliced
- Aquafaba from one bean can (bean liquid)

Directions:

1. Take a shallow bowl and add almond meal, salt
2. Pour aquafaba in another bowl, dredge avocado slices in aquafaba and then into the crumbs to get a nice coating
3. Assemble them in a single layer in your Air Fryer cooking basket, don't overlap
4. Cook for 10 minutes at 390 degrees F, give the basket a shake, and cook for 5 minutes more
5. Serve and enjoy!

Nutrition: Calories: 356 Fat: 14g Carbohydrates: 8g Protein: 23g

57. Hearty Green Beans

Preapration Time:5 Minutes

Cooking Time: 10 to 15 Minutes

Servings: 6

Ingredients:

- 1-pound green beans washed and de-stemmed
- One lemon
- Pinch of salt
- ¼ teaspoon oil

Directions:

1. Add beans to your Air Fryer cooking basket
2. Squeeze a few drops of lemon
3. Season with salt and pepper
4. Drizzle olive oil on top
5. Cook for 10-12 minutes at 400 degrees F
6. Once done, serve and enjoy!

Nutrition: Calories: 84 Fat: 5g Carbohydrates: 7g Protein: 2g

58. Parmesan Cabbage Wedges

Preapration Time: 5 Minutes

Cooking Time: 20 Minutes

Servings: 4

Ingredients:

- ½ a head cabbage
- 2 cups parmesan
- Four tablespoons melted butter
- Salt and pepper to taste

Directions:

1. Preheat your Air Fryer to 380-degree F.
2. Take a container and add melted butter, and season with salt and pepper.
3. Cover cabbages with your melted butter.
4. Coat cabbages with parmesan.
5. Transfer the coated cabbages to your Air Fryer and bake for 20 minutes.
6. Serve with cheesy sauce and enjoy!

Nutrition: Calories: 108 Fat: 7g Carbohydrates: 11g Protein: 2g

59. Extreme Zucchini Fries

Preapration Time:10 Minutes

Cooking Time: 15 to 20 Minutes

Servings: 4

Ingredients:

- Three medium zucchinis, sliced
- Two egg whites
- ½ cup seasoned almond meal
- Two tablespoons grated parmesan cheese
- ¼ teaspoon garlic powder

Directions:

1. Pre-heat your Fryer to 425-degree F.
2. Take the Air Fryer cooking basket and place a cooling rack.
3. Coat the rack with cooking spray.
4. Take a bowl, add egg whites, beat it well, and season with some pepper and salt.
5. Take another bowl and add garlic powder, cheese, and almond meal
6. Take the Zucchini sticks and dredge them in the egg and finally breadcrumbs.
7. Transfer the Zucchini to your cooking basket and spray a bit of oil.
8. Bake for 20 minutes and serve with Ranch sauce.
9. Enjoy!

Nutrition: Calories: 367 Fat: 28g Carbohydrates: 5g Protein: 4g

60. Easy Fried Tomatoes

Preapration Time:5 Minutes

Cooking Time: 10 Minutes

Servings: 3

Ingredients:

- One green tomato
- ¼ tablespoon Creole seasoning
- Salt and pepper to taste
- ¼ cup almond flour
- ½ cup buttermilk

Directions:

1. Add flour to your plate and take another plate and add buttermilk
2. Cut tomatoes and season with salt and pepper
3. Make a mix of creole seasoning and crumbs
4. Take tomato slice and cover with flour, place in buttermilk and then into crumbs
5. Repeat with all tomatoes
6. Preheat your fryer to 400-degree F
7. Cook the tomato slices for 5 minutes
8. Serve with basil and enjoy!

Nutrition: Calories: 166 Fat: 12g Carbohydrates: 11g Protein: 3g

Lightning Source UK Ltd.
Milton Keynes UK
UKHW021840170621
385713UK00002B/412